LUPUS CURE

A guide book on things one should know on proper treatment of lupus

Dr Rowan Theo

LUPUS CURE

Lupus is a chronic autoimmune disease that can affect various parts of the body. It is a complex and unpredictable condition in which the immune system attacks healthy tissues and cells instead of protecting the body from foreign invaders like viruses and bacteria. This results in inflammation and damage to multiple organs, including the skin, joints, kidneys, heart, lungs, and brain. It is a life-long condition that can be managed, but currently, there is no cure for lupus.

There are four main types of lupus: systemic lupus erythematosus (SLE), discoid lupus erythematosus (DLE), drug-induced lupus, and neonatal lupus. SLE is the most common and severe form, affecting around 70% of people with lupus. It can impact different parts of the body and cause various symptoms, making it a challenging condition to diagnose and treat.

The exact cause of lupus is unknown, but it is believed to be a combination of genetic, environmental, and hormonal factors. Research suggests that genetic predisposition plays a significant role in the development of lupus. That means that people with a family history of lupus are at a higher risk of developing the disease. Hormonal factors also influence the disease, and it is seen to affect women more than men, especially during their childbearing years. Moreover, environmental factors like infections, certain medications, and exposure to ultraviolet light can trigger lupus in susceptible individuals.

One of the hallmark signs of lupus is inflammation, which is triggered by the immune system's overactivity. Normally, when we get sick, our immune system produces antibodies and white blood cells to fight off the infection. In lupus, the immune system becomes confused and loses the ability to differentiate between healthy cells and foreign invaders. This leads to the production of autoantibodies, which attack and damage healthy tissues and organs. Over time, this chronic inflammation can cause significant damage and scarring, leading to various symptoms and complications.

The symptoms of lupus can vary from person to person and can range from mild to severe. The most common symptoms include joint pain, swelling, and stiffness, as well as fatigue, fever, and skin rashes. As the disease progresses, it can also affect internal organs, leading to complications like kidney failure, heart disease, and neurological problems. This is one of the reasons why early diagnosis and treatment are crucial in managing lupus and preventing long-term complications.

Unfortunately, lupus is often referred to as the "great imitator" because its symptoms can be similar to other conditions, making it challenging to diagnose. There are no specific tests for lupus, and the diagnosis is based on a combination of symptoms, physical examination, and certain blood tests. These tests check for the presence of autoantibodies, as well as levels of inflammation and organ functioning. Some people may also undergo additional imaging tests, such as X-rays, ultrasounds, or CT scans, to identify any damage to internal organs.

Although there is currently no cure for lupus, various treatments can help manage its symptoms and prevent flare-ups. Treatment typically includes a combination of medications, lifestyle modifications, and regular follow-up with healthcare providers. Nonsteroidal anti-inflammatory drugs (NSAIDs) can help manage joint pain and inflammation. Corticosteroids and immunosuppressants are also prescribed to suppress an overactive immune system and prevent damage to organs. It is essential for people with lupus to protect their skin from exposure to ultraviolet (UV) light, as it can trigger flare-ups. Therefore, wearing sunscreen and protective clothing, and avoiding the sun during peak hours, is crucial to managing the disease.

Types

1. Systemic Lupus Erythematosus (SLE):

SLE is the most common type of lupus, accounting for about 70% of lupus cases. It is a systemic disease, meaning it can affect any part of the body. SLE occurs when the body's immune system mistakenly attacks healthy tissues and organs, leading to inflammation and damage. It can cause a variety of symptoms, including fever, joint pain, skin rashes, fatigue, and organ damage. SLE can also involve major organs such as the heart, lungs, kidneys, and brain, making it a potentially life-threatening illness.

2. Cutaneous Lupus:

Cutaneous lupus is a type of lupus that affects the skin and is characterized by various forms of skin rashes. It can occur in people who have SLE or as a standalone condition known as discoid lupus erythematosus (DLE). The most common form of skin lupus is DLE, which causes red, scaly patches on the skin that can leave scars if not treated. Other forms of cutaneous lupus include subacute cutaneous lupus erythematosus (SCLE), lupus panniculitis, and lupus profundus, all of which cause different skin manifestations. Skin lupus rarely affects internal organs and is typically not associated with major organ involvement.

3. Drug-induced Lupus:

Drug-induced lupus is a type of lupus caused by certain medications. It is similar to SLE in terms of symptoms, but the trigger is a specific medication rather than the body's immune system. Certain drugs, such as procainamide, hydralazine, and isoniazid, have been linked to the development of drug-induced lupus. The symptoms of drug-induced lupus often subside once the culprit medication is stopped, and unlike SLE, it rarely leads to major organ damage.

4. Neonatal Lupus:

Neonatal lupus is a rare type of lupus that affects babies born to mothers with lupus or certain antibodies. It is not technically a form of lupus but is a condition caused by the transfer of maternal antibodies to the fetus during pregnancy. These antibodies can cause a variety of symptoms in newborns, including skin rashes, liver problems, and low blood cell counts. Most infants with neonatal lupus do not have long-term health effects, and the symptoms typically resolve within a few months of birth.

5. Overlap Syndrome:

Overlap syndrome, also known as mixed connective tissue disease (MCTD), is a type of lupus that shares the features of multiple autoimmune diseases, including systemic lupus, scleroderma, and polymyositis. It is characterized by a broad range of symptoms, including joint pain, skin rashes, muscle inflammation, and lung and heart involvement. The cause of overlap syndrome is unclear, but it is believed to be a combination of genetic and environmental factors. Treatment for this type of lupus usually involves a combination of medications used for the different overlapping conditions.

SYMPTOMS

1. Fatigue

Fatigue is a common symptom experienced by those with lupus. It is not just regular tiredness, but an overwhelming feeling of exhaustion that can interfere with daily activities. This fatigue is often accompanied by weakness, making it challenging to perform even simple tasks.

2. Joint pain and swelling

Joint pain and swelling are common symptoms of lupus and are often the first sign of the disease. The pain can be mild to severe and can affect any joint in the body, but it most commonly affects the hands, wrists, and knees. Joint pain can also be accompanied by stiffness, making it difficult to move the joints.

3. Skin rashes

Many people with lupus develop rashes on their skin, which can range from mild to severe. One of the most common rashes is the butterfly rash, which appears on the cheeks and nose and resembles the shape of a butterfly. Other types of rashes that may occur include scaly red patches, raised or thickened patches, and a sunburn-like rash.

4. Fever

Fever is a common symptom in lupus and is often accompanied by other flu-like symptoms such as chills, headaches, and muscle aches. The fever is usually low-grade, but in some cases, it can spike to high temperatures.

5. Photosensitivity

Many people with lupus are sensitive to sunlight and other sources of ultraviolet (UV) light.

Exposure to these UV rays can cause rashes, flare-ups, and other skin symptoms in people with lupus. Additionally, it can also trigger other symptoms such as joint pain, fatigue, and fever.

6. Hair loss

Hair loss is a common symptom of lupus, and it can occur on the scalp or other areas of the body. In some cases, the hair may grow back, but it may also become thin and brittle. In severe cases, hair loss can also lead to bald patches.

7. Mouth and nose ulcers

Around 80% of people with lupus may experience mouth ulcers, also known as oral ulcers. These are usually small and painless, but they can cause discomfort while eating or talking. Nose ulcers are less common but can be a sign of more severe disease activity.

8. Raynaud's phenomenon

Raynaud's phenomenon is a condition in which the blood vessels in the fingers and toes constrict in response to cold temperatures or stress, leading to numbness, tingling, and color changes in the affected areas. It is a common symptom of lupus and can also occur on its own.

9. Chest pain

Chest pain is a common symptom in lupus and can be caused by inflammation in the heart or the lungs. This chest pain is usually sharp and can be worsened by taking deep breaths. In severe cases, it can also lead to difficulty breathing.

10. Kidney problems

Kidney involvement is common in lupus, and it can range from mild to severe. This can lead to various symptoms, including swelling in the legs, foamy or bloody urine, high blood pressure, and changes in urination patterns.

11. Neurological symptoms

Lupus can also affect the nervous system, leading to various neurological symptoms such as headaches, dizziness, seizures, and changes in behavior and mood.

12. Gastrointestinal issues

Many people with lupus may experience gastrointestinal symptoms such as nausea, vomiting, diarrhea, and loss of appetite. These symptoms can be caused by the disease itself or as a side effect of medications used to treat lupus.

Current Treatment Measures for Lupus

The treatment of lupus is aimed at controlling the symptoms and preventing disease flares, as well as protecting the organs and tissues from damage. Treatment plans are individualized for each patient, considering their symptoms, medical history, and overall health. The most common treatment measures for lupus include medications, lifestyle changes, and regular monitoring.

Medications are the mainstay of treatment for lupus. The type of medication prescribed depends on the severity of symptoms and which part of the body is affected. The following are some of the commonly used medications for lupus:

1. Nonsteroidal anti-inflammatory drugs (NSAIDs): These are used to relieve joint pain and stiffness in lupus patients. Examples include ibuprofen, naproxen, and aspirin.

2. Antimalarials: These medications are typically used to

treat malaria but have been found to be effective in managing lupus symptoms, especially skin rashes and joint pain. The most commonly prescribed antimalarial for lupus is hydroxychloroquine.

3. Corticosteroids: These medications work by suppressing the overactive immune system in lupus patients. They are commonly used for severe symptoms or flares and can be given in the form of pills, injections, or creams. Examples include prednisone,

hydrocortisone, and dexamethasone.

4. Immunosuppressants: Similar to corticosteroids, immunosuppressants also work by suppressing the immune system to prevent it from attacking the body's own tissues. They are used for more severe cases of lupus, and examples include azathioprine, cyclophosphamide, and mycophenolate mofetil.

5. Monoclonal antibodies: These are newer medications that specifically target certain cells or

proteins involved in the immune system. For example, belimumab targets a protein called B-lymphocyte stimulator, which is overproduced in lupus patients. These medications are usually reserved for refractory cases of lupus and are given intravenously.

Apart from medications, lifestyle changes can also play a significant role in managing lupus. Patients are advised to avoid triggers that can worsen symptoms, such as stress, smoking, and excessive sunlight exposure. A healthy diet, regular exercise, and adequate rest and sleep are also essential for managing lupus.

Regular monitoring is crucial for lupus patients to ensure that the treatment plan is effective and any potential side effects are identified and managed promptly. Patients may need to undergo regular blood tests, imaging studies, and consultations with their healthcare team to monitor their disease activity and response to treatment.

In addition to these conventional treatment measures, there are also alternative and complementary therapies that have gained popularity among lupus patients. These include acupuncture, massage therapy, and dietary supplements such as fish oil and turmeric. While some patients may find these therapies helpful in managing their symptoms, it is essential to consult with a healthcare professional before trying any alternative treatment.

In recent years, there have been significant advancements in the treatment of lupus, particularly with the introduction of new medications that target specific parts of the immune system. However, there is still a need for more effective and safer treatments, as well as a cure for this chronic disease.

Medications

1. Nonsteroidal anti-inflammatory drugs (NSAIDs)

NSAIDs, such as aspirin, ibuprofen, and naproxen, are commonly used to treat pain, swelling, and inflammation associated with lupus. They work by blocking the production of prostaglandins, which are substances that contribute to inflammation and pain. These medications can also help reduce fever and stiffness in joints. However, long-term use of NSAIDs can cause side effects such as stomach ulcers, so they should be used with caution.

2. Corticosteroids

Corticosteroids, such as prednisone and methylprednisolone, are powerful anti-inflammatory drugs that can be used to control severe symptoms of lupus. They work by suppressing the immune system and reducing inflammation. Corticosteroids can be taken orally, injected, or applied topically, depending on the type and severity of symptoms. These medications can have significant side effects, including weight gain, high blood pressure, osteoporosis, and increased risk of infections. Therefore, they are usually prescribed in low doses and for short periods of time.

3. Antimalarial drugs

Chloroquine and hydroxychloroquine are commonly used antimalarial drugs that have been found to be effective in treating skin rashes, joint pain, and fatigue associated with lupus. These medications work by suppressing the immune system and reducing inflammation. They may also have additional benefits, such as reducing the risk of blood clots and protecting against damage to the heart and blood vessels. However, these medications can have side effects such as visual disturbances and gastrointestinal upset.

4. Immunosuppressants

Immunosuppressants, such as azathioprine, methotrexate, and cyclophosphamide, are often used in more severe cases of lupus where other medications have not been effective. These medications work by suppressing the immune system and reducing inflammation. They are usually prescribed in combination with other medications to help control symptoms and prevent complications. However, they can have significant side effects, including increased risk of infections and liver or kidney damage.

5. Biological therapies

Biological therapies, such as rituximab and belimumab, target specific components of the immune system that are involved in the development of lupus. These medications work by blocking the action of B cells, which produce antibodies that attack the body's own tissues. They can be effective in treating lupus symptoms and reducing the frequency of flares. However, they can also increase the risk of infections and may have other potential side effects, such as infusion reactions.

6.   Nonsteroidal immunomodulators

Nonsteroidal immunomodulators, such as thalidomide and

lenalidomide, are a newer class of medications that work by modifying the immune response. They are typically used to treat rashes and skin lesions associated with lupus. These medications can have significant side effects, including nerve damage, birth defects, and increased risk of blood clots.

7. Benlysta (belimumab)

Benlysta is the first and only medication approved specifically for the treatment of lupus. It is a biological therapy that works by targeting a protein that is believed to play a role in the development of lupus. It is approved for use in adults with active systemic lupus erythematosus (SLE) who are receiving standard therapy. Benlysta has been found to be effective in reducing the frequency of flares and improving overall symptoms, but it can also have side effects such as increased risk of infections and infusion reactions.

Lupus chance elements

Certain businesses can be at a better chance of growing lupus. Examples of chance elements for lupus encompass:

• Sex: Women are much more likely to broaden lupus than guys, however the disorder can gift as extra extreme in guys.

• Age: While lupus can arise at any age, it's most customarily identified in humans among the a long time of 15 and 44.

• Race or ethnicity: Lupus is extra common in positive ethnic businesses, including African American, Hispanic, Asian

American, Native American, or Pacific Islander

• Family records: Having a own circle of relatives records of lupus manner which you're at a extra chance of growing the situation.

Remember that having chance elements for lupus doesn't imply you'll get lupus. It simply manner which you're at accelerated chance in comparison to folks that don't have chance elements.

☐

Is lupus curable?

Currently, there's no treatment for lupus. However, there are numerous exclusive forms of remedies that permit you to manipulate your signs.

Treatment for lupus makes a specialty of numerous elements:

• treating lupus signs if you have them

• stopping lupus flares from occurring

• lowering the quantity of harm that takes place in your joints and organs

Following your healthcare company's endorsed remedy routine is critical in supporting you to manipulate your signs and to stay a regular, gratifying existence.

Healthcare companies and scientists hold their studies to higher apprehend lupus and broaden new remedies for the situation.

Lupus remedy

While there's presently no treatment for lupus at this time, medicinal drugs are to be had that will help you to manipulate your lupus signs and save you lupus flares. Your healthcare company will don't forget your lupus signs and their severity while recommending lupus remedies.

It's critical which you see your healthcare company on a ordinary basis. This lets in them to higher display your situation and decide in case your remedy plan is operating to manipulate your signs.

Additionally, your lupus signs can extrade through the years. Because of this, your healthcare company might also additionally extrade your medicinal drugs or modify the dosage of modern remedy.

In addition to remedy, your healthcare company may additionally advise life-style adjustments to assist manipulate your lupus signs. These can encompass matters including:

• warding off extra publicity to ultraviolet (UV) light

• consuming a healthful diet

• taking dietary supplements that could assist to lessen signs, including nutrition D, calcium, and fish oil

• getting ordinary exercise

• quitting smoking, in case you smoke

Lupus diet

Healthcare companies haven't set up a particular lupus diet. In general, goal to devour a healthful, well-balanced diet. This can encompass matters like:

• fish excessive in omega-three fatty acids, including salmon, tuna, or mackerel, which intake of ought to be monitored because of the want in order to be aware about multiplied mercury degrees

• ingredients excessive in calcium, including low-fats dairy products

• consuming whole-grain carbohydrate sources

• consuming a mix of colourful end result and vegetables

There also are a few ingredients that people with lupus ought to commonly keep away from, often because of the medicinal drugs they usually take. Some examples of ingredients to live far from encompass:

• Alcohol: Alcohol can engage negatively with many medicinal drugs. For instance, it is able to purpose gastrointestinal bleeding in humans taking NSAIDs. It also can growth the opportunity of irritation.

• Alfalfa: The amino acid called L-canavanine determined in alfalfa sprouts and seeds might also additionally growth irritation and result in lupus flares.

• Foods excessive in salt and cholesterol:Not handiest is reducing returned on those useful to your usual fitness, however it additionally enables to save you bloating and will increase in blood strain because of corticosteroid use.

Additionally, in case you enjoy photosensitivity because of your lupus, you can lack nutrition D. Taking a nutrition D complement might also additionally assist. You can store for nutrition D dietary supplements .

FOODS TO AVIOD

1. Foods high in saturated and trans fats

Foods that are high in saturated and trans fats, such as red meat, processed meats, fried foods, and full-fat dairy products, can increase inflammation in the body. This can worsen the symptoms of lupus, including joint pain and fatigue. These types of fats are also linked to an increased risk of heart disease, which is a common comorbidity in lupus patients. Therefore, it is recommended to limit the consumption of these foods and opt for healthier sources of fat, such as fish, avocados, and nuts.

2. Gluten

Gluten is a protein found in wheat, barley, and rye. It can trigger inflammation in people with celiac disease, an autoimmune disorder that affects the small intestines. However, recent studies suggest that gluten may also contribute to inflammation in patients with other autoimmune diseases, including lupus. Therefore, individuals with lupus may benefit from avoiding or reducing gluten in their diet. Gluten-free alternatives, such as quinoa, brown rice, and gluten-free bread, can be healthier and less inflammatory options.

3. Nightshade vegetables

Tomatoes, potatoes, eggplants, and peppers are all examples of nightshade vegetables that contain a chemical called solanine. This compound can worsen inflammation in some people, including those with autoimmune diseases like lupus. However, more research is needed to confirm this link, and some people with lupus may be able to tolerate these vegetables without any issues. If you notice an increase in symptoms after consuming nightshade vegetables, it may be best to avoid them or limit their consumption.

4. Alcohol

Alcohol consumption can have a negative impact on the symptoms of lupus. It can trigger flare-ups, worsen fatigue and joint pain, and interact with medication. Also, many medications prescribed to treat lupus can cause liver damage. Therefore, it is essential to limit alcohol consumption or avoid it altogether if you have lupus.

5. Added sugars

Foods and drinks that are high in added sugars, such as sodas, candies, and baked goods, can trigger inflammation in the body. These sugars can also lead to weight gain, which can worsen joint pain and other symptoms of lupus. Moreover, high sugar consumption has been linked to an increased risk of heart disease, which is a common comorbidity in patients with lupus. It is best to limit the intake of added sugars and choose natural sources of sweetness, such as fruits and honey, instead.

6. Excess salt

People with lupus are at a higher risk of developing high blood pressure, and consuming excess salt can worsen this condition. High blood pressure can put extra strain on the heart and blood vessels, increasing the risk of heart disease. It can also contribute to fluid retention, which can worsen swelling in the joints, commonly seen in lupus patients. Therefore, it is recommended to limit sodium intake and opt for low-sodium alternatives.

7. Oxalate-rich foods

Oxalates are compounds found in many healthy foods, such as spinach, beets, and almonds. These compounds can contribute to inflammation in the body, and some studies suggest that they may play a role in the development of kidney stones, which is a common complication of lupus. While it is essential to consume a variety of healthy foods, people with lupus may benefit from limiting their intake of oxalate-rich foods and opting for lower oxalate alternatives.

FOODS TO EAT

1. Anti-inflammatory fruits and vegetables: Due to the inflammatory nature of lupus, it is important to include plenty of anti-inflammatory foods in your diet. Fruits and vegetables such as berries, leafy greens, cruciferous vegetables, and tomatoes are excellent sources of antioxidants and vitamins that can help reduce inflammation and disease activity.

2. Omega-3 rich foods: Omega-3 fatty acids have been found to have anti-inflammatory properties and can help alleviate symptoms

of lupus. Foods such as fish (salmon, tuna, mackerel), flax seeds, chia seeds, and walnuts are great sources of omega-3s.

3. Whole grains: Whole grains are an important source of fiber and nutrients, and they also have a low glycemic index which means they won't spike your blood sugar levels. This is important for people with lupus as they are at a higher risk for developing diabetes.

4. Lean protein: Protein is essential for repairing and building tissues and maintaining a

healthy immune system. When dealing with lupus, it is important to choose lean protein sources such as chicken, turkey, fish, tofu, and beans instead of red meat.

5. Healthy fats: Healthy fats, such as olive oil, avocado, and nuts, should be included in a lupus diet. These fats can help reduce inflammation and promote heart health.

6. Calcium-rich foods: People with lupus are at a higher risk for developing osteoporosis, so it is important to include calcium-rich

foods in their diet. Dairy products, leafy greens, fortified cereals, and calcium-fortified soy products are great sources of calcium.

7. Vitamin D sources: Vitamin D plays an important role in maintaining bone health and immune function. People with lupus are at a higher risk of vitamin D deficiency, so it is important to include foods such as fatty fish, eggs, and fortified foods in their diet. Sun exposure is also a natural source of vitamin D.

8. Green tea: Green tea contains polyphenols, which have anti-inflammatory properties and may help reduce the severity of lupus symptoms. It is also a good alternative to caffeinated beverages, which can trigger lupus flares.

9. Garlic: Garlic has been used for its medicinal properties for centuries, and it may also help with lupus symptoms. Studies have shown that garlic has anti-inflammatory and immune-modulating effects, making it a beneficial addition to a lupus diet.

10. Probiotic-rich foods: Probiotics can help improve gut health and boost the immune system. People with lupus are at a higher risk for gut-related issues, so incorporating probiotic-rich foods such as yogurt, kefir, sauerkraut, and kimchi can help improve symptoms.

11. Turmeric: Turmeric contains a compound called curcumin, which has anti-inflammatory and antioxidant properties. Adding turmeric to your diet may help

reduce inflammation and improve joint pain associated with lupus.

12. Ginger: Ginger has been used for centuries to treat various inflammatory conditions. Its anti-inflammatory properties may also help with managing lupus symptoms. Ginger can be added to meals or consumed as a tea.

13. Dark chocolate: Dark chocolate contains antioxidants called flavonoids, which can help reduce inflammation and have been shown to improve cognitive function. Choose high-quality dark

chocolate with at least 70% cocoa to reap the health benefits.

14. Citrus fruits: Vitamin C is an important nutrient for people with lupus as it helps boost the immune system and may have anti-inflammatory effects. Citrus fruits, such as oranges, grapefruits, and lemons, are excellent sources of vitamin C.

15. Water: Staying hydrated is crucial for overall health and managing lupus symptoms. Drinking enough water can help flush out toxins and prevent

dehydration, which can worsen lupus symptoms.

EXERCISES TO DO

Here are some exercises that may help those with Lupus:

1. Low-impact aerobic exercises

Low-impact aerobic exercises, such as swimming, walking, and cycling, are recommended for people with Lupus. These exercises help to improve cardiovascular health, strengthen muscles, and increase flexibility without putting too much stress on the joints. They also help to increase endurance and reduce fatigue, which is a common symptom of Lupus.

2. Stretching

Stretching is important for maintaining flexibility and range of motion in the joints. People with Lupus may experience stiffness and pain in their joints, so stretching helps to loosen up tight muscles and improve mobility. It is important to do gentle stretches and avoid over-stretching, which can cause injury.

3. Yoga

Yoga is a combination of stretching, breathing, and relaxation techniques that can be beneficial for people with Lupus. It helps to improve flexibility, balance, and muscle strength, while also promoting relaxation and reducing stress. However, it is important to choose gentle and modified yoga poses that do not put too much strain on the joints.

4. Pilates

Pilates is a low-impact exercise that focuses on strengthening the core muscles and improving posture. It can be beneficial for people with Lupus who may experience muscle weakness and joint pain. However, it is important to consult with a certified Pilates instructor who can modify the exercises to suit your specific needs.

5. Water exercises

Exercising in the water, such as swimming or water aerobics, is a great option for people with Lupus. The buoyancy of the water helps to reduce the impact on the joints, while also providing resistance to strengthen muscles. Water exercises can also be beneficial for people with joint pain as it helps to reduce inflammation and swelling.

6. Resistance training

Resistance or strength training is important for building and maintaining muscle strength. This type of exercise can help to improve joint stability and prevent the loss of muscle mass, which is common in people with Lupus. However, it is important to start with light weights and gradually increase as you gain strength.

7. Tai Chi

Tai Chi is a low-impact exercise that originated in China and combines slow, gentle movements with breathing techniques. It can be beneficial for people with Lupus to improve balance, flexibility, and muscle strength. Additionally, it promotes relaxation and stress reduction.

8. Cycling

Cycling is a low-impact exercise that can be done indoors or outdoors. It is a great way to strengthen the leg muscles, improve cardiovascular health, and reduce stress. It can be beneficial for people with Lupus who experience joint pain, as it puts less stress on the joints compared to other forms of exercise.

9. Resistance band exercises

Resistance bands are a great option for people with Lupus as they provide resistance to strengthen muscles without putting too much strain on the joints. They are also lightweight and portable, making it easy to do exercises at home or while traveling.

10. Dancing

Dancing is a fun and enjoyable form of exercise that can benefit both physical and mental health. It can help to improve balance, coordination, flexibility, and cardiovascular health. People with Lupus can choose low-impact forms of dancing, such as ballroom dancing, to reduce strain on the joints.

When starting an exercise routine, it is important to consult with a doctor, physical therapist, or certified fitness professional to create a personalized plan that takes into consideration your individual needs and limitations. It is also important to listen to your body and start slowly, gradually increasing the intensity and duration of your workouts as you build strength and endurance.

Drug for lupus cure

Use of positive prescription medicinal drugs can result in drug-brought on lupus (DIL). DIL will also be known as drug-brought on lupus erythematosus.

DIL can broaden via the lengthy-time period use of positive prescribed medicinal drugs, usually after simply months of taking a drug.

There are many pills which can purpose you to broaden DIL. Some examples encompass:

• antimicrobials, including terbinafine (an antifungal) and

pyrazinamide (a tuberculosis remedy)

• anticonvulsant pills, like phenytoin(Dilantin) and valproate

• arrhythmia pills, including quinidineand procainamide

• pills for excessive blood strain, like timolol (Timoptic, Istlol) and hydroxyzine

• biologics known as anti-TNF-alpha agents, including infliximab (Remicade) and etanercept (Enbrel)

While DIL mimics the signs of SLE, in maximum instances the situation doesn't commonly have an effect on fundamental organs. However, it is able to purpose pericarditis and pleurisy. DIL commonly is going away inside weeks of preventing the drugs that prompted it to arise.

Importance of Early Diagnosis and Treatment

Early diagnosis and treatment are crucial in managing lupus and improving outcomes for patients. Here are some reasons why timely diagnosis and treatment are essential for individuals with lupus:

1. Preventing Damage to Organs

One of the most significant benefits of early diagnosis and treatment of lupus is preventing damage to the body's organs. Lupus can cause inflammation in various organs, such as the kidneys, heart, and brain, which, if left untreated, can lead to organ dysfunction and failure. With early detection and treatment, the progression of organ damage can be slowed or even halted, preventing serious complications and improving the patient's quality of life.

2. Better Management of Flare-ups

Lupus is a disease characterized by periods of flare-ups and remission. During a flare-up, the symptoms of lupus can worsen and cause significant discomfort and pain for the patient. However, with prompt treatment, the severity and duration of flare-ups can be reduced, allowing patients to better manage their symptoms and maintain their daily activities.

3. Early Prevention of Lupus Nephritis

Lupus nephritis is a severe complication of lupus where the disease attacks the kidneys, leading to inflammation and damage. It is estimated that up to

60% of people with lupus develop lupus nephritis, and it is one of the leading causes of death in lupus patients. Early diagnosis and treatment can help prevent or delay the onset of lupus nephritis, reducing the risk of complications and improving long-term outcomes for patients.

4. Improved Survival Rates

Early diagnosis and treatment of lupus have been shown to improve survival rates for patients. Research has found that patients diagnosed with lupus early on have a 90% chance of surviving for at least five years, compared to only 46% for those diagnosed at a later stage. This stark difference highlights the importance of timely detection and treatment for the long-term survival of individuals with lupus.

5. Better Control of Symptoms

Lupus can cause a wide range of symptoms, including joint pain, fatigue, skin rashes, and fever. These symptoms can be both physically and emotionally challenging for patients, affecting their daily lives and overall well-being. Early diagnosis and treatment can help control these symptoms, allowing patients to manage their disease better and live a more comfortable life.

6. Preventing Damage to Mental Health

Living with a chronic illness like lupus can take a toll on a person's mental health. The physical symptoms and the unpredictable nature of the disease can lead to anxiety, depression, and other mental health issues. Early diagnosis and treatment of lupus can help prevent or minimize the impact of the disease on a patient's mental health and improve their overall quality of life.

7. Cost-effective Treatment

Early diagnosis and treatment of lupus can also lead to significant cost savings for both the patient and the healthcare system. People with lupus often require long-term management and regular medication to control their symptoms and prevent complications. Delayed diagnosis and treatment can result in more severe disease and more expensive treatments, which can be a significant burden on patients and the healthcare system.

CONCLUSION

In conclusion, lupus is a complex and unpredictable autoimmune disease that affects millions of people globally. Despite extensive research and medical advancement, there is currently no known cure for lupus. However, there have been significant developments in managing the symptoms and improving the quality of life for those living with the disease.

One of the major challenges in finding a cure for lupus is its complexity. Lupus can affect multiple organs and systems in the body, making it difficult to identify a single target for treatment. Additionally, the disease presents differently in each individual, making it challenging to develop a universal cure that would work for everyone. This has led to a focus on individualized treatment plans and a combination of medications to manage the symptoms of the disease.

Another obstacle in finding a cure for lupus is the lack of understanding of its underlying causes. While it is known to be an autoimmune disease, the exact trigger for the immune system attacking healthy cells is still unclear. This makes it difficult to develop targeted treatments that can address the root cause of the disease. Additionally, genetics and environmental factors also play a role in the development of lupus, making it a highly complex and multifactorial disease.

Despite these challenges, there have been significant advancements in managing lupus symptoms and slowing down disease progression. Medications such as corticosteroids, immunosuppressants, and biologics have been crucial in reducing inflammation and managing symptoms such as joint pain, fatigue, and skin rashes. However, these treatments come with side effects, and long-term use can increase the risk of developing other health complications. Therefore, there is a need for more specific and targeted therapies to reduce the reliance on these medications.

One promising area of research in finding a cure for lupus is gene therapy. Scientists are exploring the use of gene manipulation to correct the faulty immune response in lupus. This involves modifying the genetic material of the immune cells to prevent them from attacking healthy cells. While this is still in the early stages of testing, it shows great potential in providing a cure for lupus in the future.

Another promising area of research is the use of stem cells. Stem cells have the ability to develop into different types of cells in the body, and researchers are exploring their potential in repairing the damaged tissues and cells caused by lupus. This could potentially reverse the damage caused by lupus and provide a permanent cure. However, more research is needed in this area, and clinical trials are ongoing to determine the safety and efficacy of this treatment option.

Aside from medical treatments, lifestyle modifications can also significantly impact the course of lupus. A balanced diet, regular exercise, and stress management can help reduce inflammation and improve overall health. It is essential for those with lupus to listen to their bodies and make necessary lifestyle changes to support their immune system.

In addition to medical and lifestyle interventions, psychological support is also crucial in managing lupus. Living with a chronic and unpredictable illness can take a toll on one's mental health, and it is vital to address this aspect of lupus management. Support groups, therapy, and counseling can help individuals cope with the emotional and psychological impact of the disease.

A cure for lupus is still elusive, but with ongoing research and advancements in medical technology, there is hope for a cure in the future. It is essential to continue supporting and investing in lupus research to better understand the disease and develop more effective treatments. In the meantime, individuals with lupus can work closely with their healthcare team to manage the symptoms and improve their quality of life. With the right management plan and support, it

is possible to live a fulfilling life
with lupus.

www.ingramcontent.com/pod-product-compliance
Lightning Source LLC
Chambersburg PA
CBHW070820280726
48660CB00016B/2145